YOUR KNOWLEDGE HAS VALUE

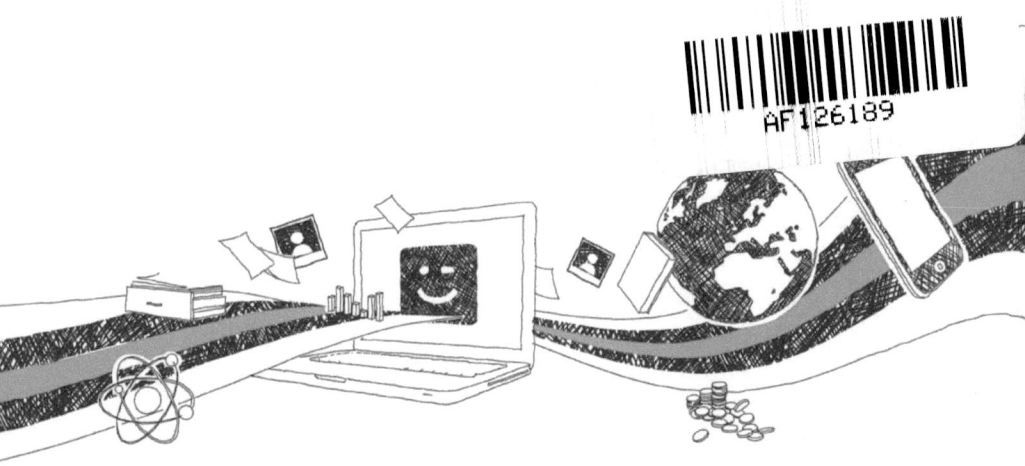
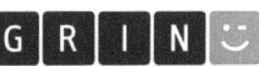

Bibliographic information published by the German National Library:

The German National Library lists this publication in the National Bibliography; detailed bibliographic data are available on the Internet at http://dnb.dnb.de .

Imprint:

Copyright © 2020 GRIN Verlag
Print and binding: Books on Demand GmbH, Norderstedt Germany
ISBN: 9783346206190

This book at GRIN:

https://www.grin.com/document/903765

Samuel Lehmann

The Effect of Strength Training on Gait for Individuals with Multiple Sclerosis

GRIN Verlag

GRIN - Your knowledge has value

Since its foundation in 1998, GRIN has specialized in publishing academic texts by students, college teachers and other academics as e-book and printed book. The website www.grin.com is an ideal platform for presenting term papers, final papers, scientific essays, dissertations and specialist books.

Visit us on the internet:

http://www.grin.com/

http://www.facebook.com/grincom

http://www.twitter.com/grin_com

The Effect of Strength Training on Gait for Individuals with Multiple Sclerosis

University: James Cook University

College: College of Healthcare Sciences

Neuroscience in Physiotherapy

Student Name: Samuel Lehmann

Contents

Characterised by the demyelination of motor and sensory axons in the central nervous system, multiple sclerosis (MS) is an autoimmune, neurodegenerative disease most commonly affecting young women (Halabchi et al., 2017). The chronic course of the disease involves either stable phases interrupted by periods of degeneration (relapsing-remitting MS) or progressive, continuous disease progression (primary and secondary progressive MS) (Callesen et al., 2018). Due to the varying progressive nature of MS and the significance of lesion location, symptom severity and experiences can range, including impaired cognition, balance and sensory deficits, spasticity, muscle weakness and fatigue (Halabchi et al., 2017).

More specifically, gait limitations were reported in 93% of people with MS (PwMS) 10 years following diagnosis, signifying the importance of rehabilitation approaches targeting gait restoration (Manago et al., 2019). Cerebellar dysfunction and lower limb muscle weakness have been identified as the primary contributing factors to gait ataxia; generally typified by reduced walking speed, shortened step length and longer stance phase in individuals with MS (Heine et al., 2018). In the past, PwMS were advised by health professionals to abstain from exercise amid concerns of triggering neurodegenerative progression and excessive fatigue (Dalgas et al., 2008). However, Halabchi et al. (2017) outlined that it has since been discovered that inactivity in MS patients leads to deconditioning, eventually resulting in the lower extremity muscle weakness partly responsible for gait impairment. It can thereby be deduced that interventions targeting muscle weakness, such as strength training (ST), serve as a promising strategy towards combatting MS gait dysfunction as a consequence of inactivity (Halabchi et al., 2017).

The suitability of a multidisciplinary approach towards MS rehabilitation is assured as the heterogenous nature of the disease complicates the possibility of a consistent, universally effective treatment strategy (Smedal et al., 2006). As a part of this approach, physiotherapy is a common, widely accepted form of MS intervention delivery proven to reduce neurodegeneration and improve functional outcomes (Smedal et al., 2006). Frequently utilised by physiotherapists, ST is recognised as an appropriate intervention for MS as the findings of numerous studies align in proving its tolerability by PwMS and effectiveness towards improving muscle strength (Dalgas et al., 2008). For instance, Heine et al. (2018) identified limited ankle push-off power as a key element reducing gait efficiency in PwMS, subsequently assigning a sample of 10 PwMS an eight-week resistance training program and detecting improvements in plantarflexion strength and gait efficiency.

Although Manago et al. (2019) along with Dalgas et al. (2008) supported the effectiveness of ST towards promoting muscle strength, they questioned its ability to improve functional outcomes, such as gait, in PwMS. This lack of consensus was mirrored by the work of Hayes et al., (2011) failing to establish a positive link between ST and gait, or even muscle strength, thereby warranting further investigation. Accordingly, the following review aimed to explore and evaluate the literature surrounding the effectiveness of ST in improving gait in PwMS.

Methodology

Study search parameters: Inclusion and exclusion criteria

A literature search was conducted on the 9th and 10th of April 2020, utilising four databases: PubMed, Scopus, Ovid and CINAHL. The title, abstract and keyword search terms entered were "("strength training" OR "resistance training") AND gait AND ("multiple sclerosis" OR "disseminated sclerosis")", with temporal restrictions set to only include articles published from 2010 to 2020 and filters applied to include peer reviewed articles. Following the initial search, duplicate publications were removed and the title and abstract of each study were screened using the inclusion and exclusion criteria. Randomised control trials or reputable case control studies surrounding the effect of ST on gait in PwMS were deemed eligible and meta-analyses, systematic reviews and studies surrounding irrelevant populations, interventions or outcomes were excluded. The remaining articles were then screened in full-text form and further refined to exclude those with combined interventions, absence of a comparison group, lack of full-text availability or published in a language other than English.

Data collection

Once the search refinement was complete, the articles' sample selection, interventions, outcomes and main findings were extracted and tabulated. The findings and conclusions of each study, along with their reputability, were then compared and critically analysed in order to reach a substantiated conclusion.

Results

An initial literature search surfaced 92 articles from the selected databases. The search

refinement was completed and displayed in accordance with the PRISMA (Preferred Reporting

Items for Systematic Reviews and Meta-Analyses) flow diagram, as shown in figure 1 (Moher

et al., 2009). Following the removal of duplicates, 58 publications remained. Title and abstract

screening facilitated the further exclusion of 48 studies in line with the inclusion and exclusion

criteria. 10 articles were then screened in full; five were excluded due to combined

interventions and one due to the lack of a comparison group. The remaining four studies were

deemed suitable and data extraction involved the tabulation of the authors, study designs,

sample populations, interventions, outcomes, statistical analyses and conclusions of each study,

shown in table 1.

PRISMA 2009 Flow Diagram

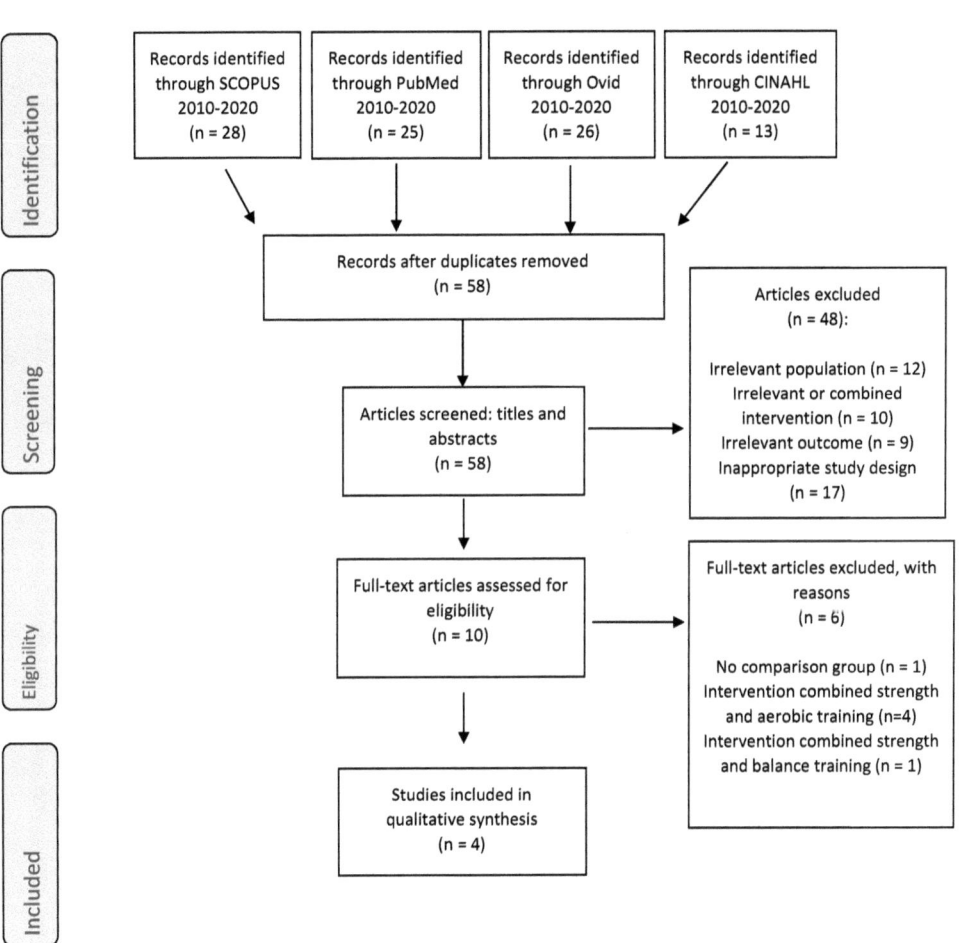

Figure 1. PRISMA flow diagram detailing literature search and selection (Moher et al., 2009)

Table 1: Data collection

Authors & Publication Date	Study Design	Sample Allocation, Disability Level	Intervention	Measurement	P-value & Statistical Analysis Test	Outcomes/Results	Conclusions
Braendvik et al. 2015	Single blinded randomised parallel group trial	ST: n = 15, EDSS score 3.2 ± 1.4 TT: n = 11, EDSS score 3.1 ± 1.6 *All MS patients	ST: Leg press, knee ext, ankle pf, ankle df, hip abd, 2 sets 6 reps, 80% 1RM, 3x/wk, 8wks TT: Walking at preferred speed with inc slope, walking with verbal guidance, walking at 10-40% preferred speed inc, each 7 min, 3x/wk, 8wks	FAP, WWE, APaccRMS, VaccRMS, MLaccRMS	ANCOVA, paired samples t-tests and Wilcoxon signed ranked test α = 0.05	TT group saw a nearly significant improvement in FAP score (3.2a.u., p = 0.051) and a significant reduction in WWE (-1.43ml/kg, p = 0.025). ST group saw no significant gait improvements	TT was superior to ST in improving gait outcomes, such as walking ability, energy expenditure and balance control in PwMS
Callesen et al. 2019	Randomised controlled multi-centre trial	PRT: n = 23, EDSS score 4 BMCT: n = 20, EDSS score 4 Control: n = 28, EDSS score 3.5 *All MS patients with SSST score > 8 sec or T25FW > 5 sec	PRT: Leg press, knee ext, knee flex, hip flex, hip ext, 3-4 sets 8-12 reps, 8-15RM, 2x/wk, 10 wks BMCT: 5min sitting, 5min standing, 10min stepping, 2x10min walking, 10 min eye-movement training, 2x/wk, 10 wks Control: Usual care and PA level. PRT + BMCT after 10wks	T25FW, SSST, MSWS, 6MWT	ANOVA, Kruskal-Wallis test and Chi-square test α = 0.05	BMCT group significantly improved T25FW test (.10m/s, p = .04), SSST (-2.25sec, p < .01) and MSWS (-7.3a.u., p = .01) compared to the control group. PRT group saw no significant gait improvements	BMCT, but not PRT, significantly improved short distance, complex and regular gait in PwMS
Dodd et al. 2011	Single blinded randomised controlled trial	PRT: n = 36 Control: n = 35 *All RRMS patients with AI scores of 2, 3 or 4	PRT: Leg press, reverse leg press, knee flex, knee ext, calf raise, 2 sets 10-12 reps, 10-12RM, 2x/week, 10 wks Control: Usual care and a social program	2MWT, FWS	ANCOVA α = 0.05	PRT group did not significantly increase 2MWT score (2.8m) or FWS (.05m/s) in comparison with the control group	PRT did not improve gait performance in PwMS
Manca et al. 2020	Randomised controlled pilot trial	DST: n = 13, EDSS score 3.3 ± .89 CST: n = 12, EDSS score 4 ± 1.42 *All RRMS patients with inter-side difference in ankle df of strength ≥ 20%	ST intervention for both groups involved high-intensity isokinetic concentric training, 3 sets 4 maximal efforts, 3x/wk, 6 wks DST: Most-affected ankle dorsiflexors trained CST: Least-affected ankle dorsiflexors trained	Participants walked 10m barefoot and gait data was collected using a stereo-photogrammetric system	ANOVA and ANCOVA α = 0.05	DST group significantly increased walking speed (0.14m/s < .0001), cadence (8.1strides/min, p = 0.003) and stride length (.07m, p = .04) and significantly reduced stride time (-.09s, p < 0.03). CST group saw no significant gait improvements	DST, but not CST, of the ankle dorsiflexors significantly improved gait performance in PwMS

Notes: EDSS scores are recorded as mean ± SD, Results are recorded as (pre-post change, p-value)

Abbreviations: abd, abduction; α, alpha value; AI, ambulation index; ANOVA, analysis of variance; ANCOVA, analysis of covariance; APaccRMS, anteroposterior acceleration root mean square; a.u., arbitrary unit; BMCT, balance and motor control training; CST, contralateral strength training; df, dorsiflexion; DST, direct strength training; EDSS, Expanded Disability Status Scale; ext, extension; FAP, Functional Ambulation Profile; flex, flexion; FWS, fast walking speed; inc, increased; MLaccRMS, mediolateral acceleration root mean square; min, minutes; MSWS, Multiple Sclerosis Walking Scale; pf, plantarflexion; PRT, progressive resistance training; reps, repetitions; RM, repetition maximum; RRMS, relapsing-remitting multiple sclerosis; sec, seconds; SSST, Six Step Spot Test; SD, standard deviation; ST, strength training; TT, treadmill training; T25FW, Timed 25 Foot Walk; VaccRMS, vertical acceleration root mean square; wk, week; WWE, walking work economy; 2MWT, 2 Minute Walk Test; 6MWT, 6 Minute Walk Test.

Discussion

Following the evaluation of each study, it was identified that the specific effects of ST on gait in PwMS varied, but generally followed a trend of ineffectiveness. Brændvik et al. (2015) uncovered that treadmill training was superior to ST in improving gait outcomes. This was supported by Callesen et al., (2019) again proving the inferiority of a form of ST, progressive resistance training, (PRT) to an alternate intervention, balance and motor control training. The general ineffectiveness of ST was further reinforced by Dodd et al. (2011) as PRT again failed to improve gait outcomes compared to a control group, receiving only social care. However, confuting evidence was presented by Manca et al. (2020) as direct strength training (DST) of weakened ankle dorsiflexors induced significant gait improvements. Despite the overarching conclusive similarities, the true comparability of the results was influenced by inter-study discrepancies in gait outcome measures, ST interventions and sample population selections.

Gait outcome measures; speed, endurance and quality

The selection of outcome measures varied greatly across each study, limiting the ability to directly compare gait changes generated by ST. Accordingly, the range of outcomes can be classified as gait speed, endurance or quality to ensure comparability. Gait speed constitutes a number of measures utilised by the authors; Brændvik et al. (2015) incorporated gait speed into an arbitrary Functional Ambulant Profile (FAP) score, failing to significantly improve following ST intervention (-1.4, p = .844). Similar findings arose in the works of Callesen et al. (2019) and Dodd et al. (2011) as the PRT groups in each study saw insignificant increases in Timed 25 Foot Walk (T25FW; .02m/s, p = 0.08) and Fast Walking Speed (FWS; 0.5m/s) scores, respectively. These results are unexpected when considering that the ST interventions within each of the aforementioned studies incorporated knee flexion and extension exercises and a significant relationship has been previously identified between hamstring and quadriceps strength and gait speed (Thoumie et al., 2005). Further contradicting this, gait speed was found to significantly increase (0.14m/s, p < .0001) by Manca et al. (2020) following DST of the ankle dorsiflexors.

Gait endurance has been shown to undergo deterioration at greater rates than speed in PwMS, likely correlating with the prevalence of increased fatigue levels (Filli et al., 2018). Brændvik et al. (2015) measured gait endurance in the form of Walking Work Economy (WWE), serving as a limitation of the study as explanation of the measure's logistics, and its implications on endurance, was minimal, potentially generating interpretation bias. Therefore, it can only be assumed that ST did not improve gait endurance as WWE saw no significant improvement, (-.68kg/L, p = 0.061) with similar, more concrete results emerging from the work of Dodd et al. (2011) as PRT failed to significantly enhance Two Minute Walk Test scores (2.8m) (Brændvik et al., 2015). Likewise, Callesen et al. (2019) found no significant progression in Six Metre Walk Test scores (12.6m, p = .30) following ST intervention involving the highest training volume across all four studies, refuting previous findings eluding to a correlation between higher ST volume and improved gait endurance (Dalgas et al., 2009). Notably, the promising findings produced by Manca et al. (2020) did not extend to incorporate gait endurance, thus serving as a limitation of the conclusive ability of the study surrounding improved gait outcomes.

Similar trends found in gait speed and endurance results were also identified in terms of gait quality. Parameters such as stability and weight transfer constituted the FAP score outcome measure utilised by Brændvik et al., (2015) resulting in no significant improvements following ST intervention (-1.4, p = .844). Similar results were noted by Callesen et al. (2019) in the form of the Six Step Spot Test (-0.5sec, p = 0.52) and Multiple Sclerosis Walking Scale (-4.2, p = 0.16) as insignificant changes were recorded for both in comparison with the control group. The lack of a gait quality outcome measure highlights a limitation of the work of Dodd et al., (2011) impacting the internal validity of the study as relationships between ST and gait parameters beyond speed and endurance were not investigated. On the other hand, Manca et al. (2020) recorded significant improvements in cadence, stride length and stride time following DST of the ankle dorsiflexors; utilising three parameters previously identified as clinically relevant to PwMS, thereby deeming outcome measure selection as a strength of the study.

Interventions

Despite being based on the same fundamental principles, the adopted ST interventions were not entirely consistent across each study. The ST interventions incorporated by Brændvik et al., (2015), Callesen et al. (2019) and Dodd et al. (2011) aligned in terms of exercise selection, each involving hip and knee, flexion and extension along with ankle plantarflexion and dorsiflexion. Considering this, the failure of ST to induce significant gait improvements could be potentially attributed to a lack of training specificity and contribution to functionality, whereby task-specific ST would promote increases in strength more relevant to gait (Manago et al., 2019). The key differences separating the ST interventions were frequency, volume and intensity; previous findings eluded to intensities above 80% as optimal for gait improvement in PwMS, classifying the intensities applied in each study besides that of Manca et al., (2020) as insufficient (Dalgas et al., 2009). Furthermore, Dalgas et al. (2009) and Filipi et al. (2010) previously claimed that 12 weeks and six months, respectively, were optimal intervention period lengths in this context. However, this was strongly challenged by the results of Manca et al. (2020) as significant gait improvements were evident following only six weeks of ST.

Sample populations and study designs

Although Dodd et al. (2011) and Manca et al. (2020) only included people with relapsing-remitting MS, the sample populations recruited by each study were homogeneous in terms of disability level, measured by the Extended Disability Status Scale (EDSS) and Ambulation Index (AI). Accordingly, the external validity of the studies' findings was impacted as PwMS with greater than mild or moderate disability levels (EDSS > 6.5; AI > 4) were not involved, suggesting that future similar studies should incorporate a greater range of disability levels. This is especially endorsed on the basis that ST participation by PwMS with EDSS scores greater than 8.0 has been cleared as safe (Filipi et al., 2010).

The promising findings produced by Manca et al. (2020) were tarnished by the failure to include a control group in the study design, weakening the internal validity of the study. In addition, the multi-centre design utilised by Callesen et al. (2019) introduced the risk of variation in intervention consistency as ST machines were unlikely identical across clinics, thereby reducing internal validity while increasing external validity due to the realistic use of multiple existing clinics. However, the thoroughness and consistency of randomisation and blinding techniques throughout each study must be noted and praised, aiming to ensure internal validity.

Conclusion

Gait impairments are highly prevalent in PwMS and have been found to vary in severity and correlate with deterioration of muscle strength. Hence, ST has been regarded as a promising avenue for PwMS although its effectiveness in promoting improvements in gait were unsubstantiated. The purpose of this review was to explore and evaluate the literature surrounding the effectiveness of ST in improving gait in PwMS. Following the analysis of four studies, ST could not be confirmed as effective in improving gait; as was the case in the works of Brændvik et al., (2015) Callesen et al., (2019) and Dodd et al., (2011), although outcome measure disparities and ST intervention selections were identified as potential factors influencing the findings. However, an alternate approach utilised by Manca et al. (2020) in carrying out DST of the ankle dorsiflexors saw significant improvements in gait speed and quality. When considering the lack of supporting evidence uncovered, it can be concluded that moderate intensity ST over a period of 6-10 weeks should not be recommended clinically for the purpose of improving gait in PwMS. Future investigations should explore the effectiveness of higher intensity, task-specific ST applied over a longer intervention period to a greater range of disability levels.

References

Brændvik, S. M., Koret, T., Helbostad, J. L., Lorås, H., Bråthen, G., Hovdal, H. O., & Aamot, I. L. (2015). Treadmill Training or Progressive Strength Training to Improve Walking in People with Multiple Sclerosis? A Randomized Parallel Group Trial. *Physiotherapy Research International, 21*(4), 228-236. https://doi.org/10.1002/pri.1636

Callesen, J., Cattaneo, D., Brincks, J., & Dalgas, U. (2018). How does strength training and balance training affect gait and fatigue in patients with Multiple Sclerosis? A study protocol of a randomized controlled trial. *NeuroRehabilitation, 42*(2), 131-142. https://doi.org/ 10.3233/NRE-172238

Callesen, J., Cattaneo, D., Brincks, J., Jørgensen, M. K., & Dalgas, U. (2019). How do resistance training and balance and motor control training affect gait performance and fatigue impact in people with multiple sclerosis? A randomized controlled multi-center study. *Multiple Sclerosis Journal.* https://doi.org/10.1177/1352458519865740

Dalgas, U., Stenager, E., & Ingemann-Hansen, T. (2008). Multiple sclerosis and physical exercise: recommendations for the application of resistance-, endurance- and combined training. *Multiple Sclerosis, 14*(1), 35-53. https://doi.org/10.1177/1352458507079445

Dalgas, U., Stenager, E., Jakobsen, J., Petersen, T., Hansen, H., & Knudsen, C. (2009). Resistance training improves muscle strength and functional capacity in multiple sclerosis. *Neurology, 73*(18), 1478–1484. https://doi.org/10.1212/WNL.0b013e3181bf98b4

Dodd, K. J., Taylor, N. F., Shields, N., Prasad, D., McDonald, E., & Gillon, A. (2011).
Progressive resistance training did not improve walking but can improve muscle
performance, quality of life and fatigue in adults with multiple sclerosis: a
randomized controlled trial. *Multiple Sclerosis Journal, 17*(11), 1362-1374.
https://doi.org/10.1177/1352458511409084

Filipi, M. L., Leuschen, M. P., Huisinga, J., Schmaderer, L., Vogel, J., Kucera, D., &
Stergiou, N. (2010). Impact of Resistance Training on Balance and Gait in Multiple
Sclerosis, *International Journal of MS Care, 12*(1), 6-12.
https://doi.org/10.7224/1537-2073-12.1.6

Filli, L., Sutter, T., Easthope, C. S., Killeen, T., Meyer, C., Reuter, K., Lörincz, L., Bolliger,
M., Weller, M., Curt, A., Straumann, D., Linnebank, M., & Zörner, B. (2018).
Profiling walking dysfunction in multiple sclerosis: characterisation, classification
and progression over time. *Scientific Reports, 8*(1), 4984.
https://doi.org/10.1038/s41598-018-22676-0

Halabchi, F., Alizadeh, Z., Sahraian, M. A., & Abolhasani, M. (2017). Exercise prescription
for patients with multiple sclerosis; potential benefits and practical recommendations.
BMC Neurology, 17(1), 185. https://doi.org/10.1186/s12883-017-0960-9

Hayes, H. A., Gappmaier, E., & LaStayo, P. C. (2011). Effects of high-intensity resistance
training on strength, mobility, balance, and fatigue in individuals with multiple
sclerosis: a randomized controlled trial. *Journal of Neurologic Physical Therapy,
35*(1), 2-10. https://doi.org/10.1097/NPT.0b013e31820b5a9d

Heine, M., Richards, R., Geurtz, B., Los, F., Rietberg, M., Harlaar, J., Gerrits, K., Beckerman, H., & de Groot, V. (2018). Preliminary effectiveness of a sequential exercise intervention on gait function in ambulant patients with multiple sclerosis — A pilot study. *Clinical Biomechanics, 62*(1), 1-6. https://doi.org/10.1016/j.clinbiomech.2018.12.012

Manago, M. M., Glick, S., Hebert, J. R., Coote, S., & Schenkman, M. (2019). Strength Training to Improve Gait in People with Multiple Sclerosis A Critical Review of Exercise Parameters and Intervention Approaches, *International Journal of MS Care, 21*(2), 47-56. https://doi.org/10.7224/1537-2073.2017-079

Manca, A., Peruzzi, A., Aiello, E., Cereatti, A., Martinez, G., Deriu, F., & Della Croce, U. (2020). Gait changes following direct versus contralateral strength training: A randomized controlled pilot study in individuals with multiple sclerosis. *Gait & Posture, 78*, 13-18. https://doi.org/10.1016/j.gaitpost.2020.02.017

Moher, D., Liberati, A., Tetzlaff, J., Altman, D. G., & The PRISMA Group. (2009). Preferred Reporting Items for Systematic Reviews and Meta-Analyses: The PRISMA Statement. *PLOS Medicine, 6*(7). https://doi.org/10.1371/journal.pmed.1000097

Smedal, T., Lygren, H., Myhr, K. M., Moe-Nilssen, R., Gjelsvik, B., Gjelsvik, O., & Strand L. I. (2006). Balance and gait improved in patients with MS after physiotherapy based on the Bobath concept. *Physiotherapy Research International, 11*(2), 104-116. https://doi.org/10.1002/pri.327

Thoumie, P., Lamotte, D., Cantalloube, S., Faucher, M., & Amarenco, G. (2005). Motor determinants of gait in 100 ambulatory patients with multiple sclerosis. *Multiple Sclerosis, 11*(4), 485-491. https://doi.org/10.1191/1352458505ms1176oa

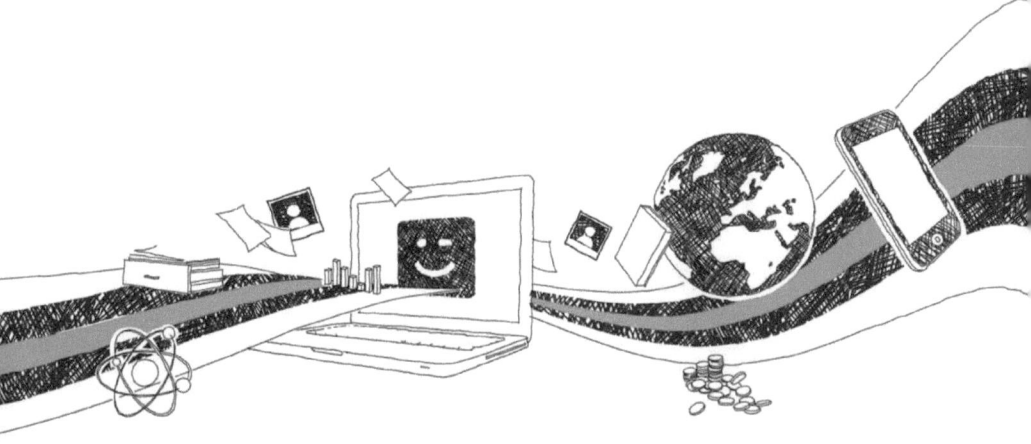
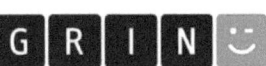